Wall Pilates

For Seniors Over 70

A Safe and Gentle Way to Build Strength, Balance, and Flexibility

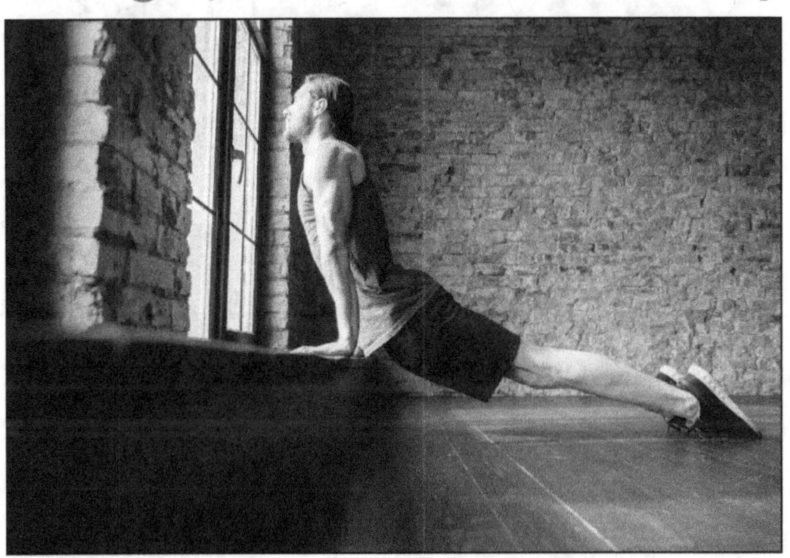

By

Taylor Susan. C.

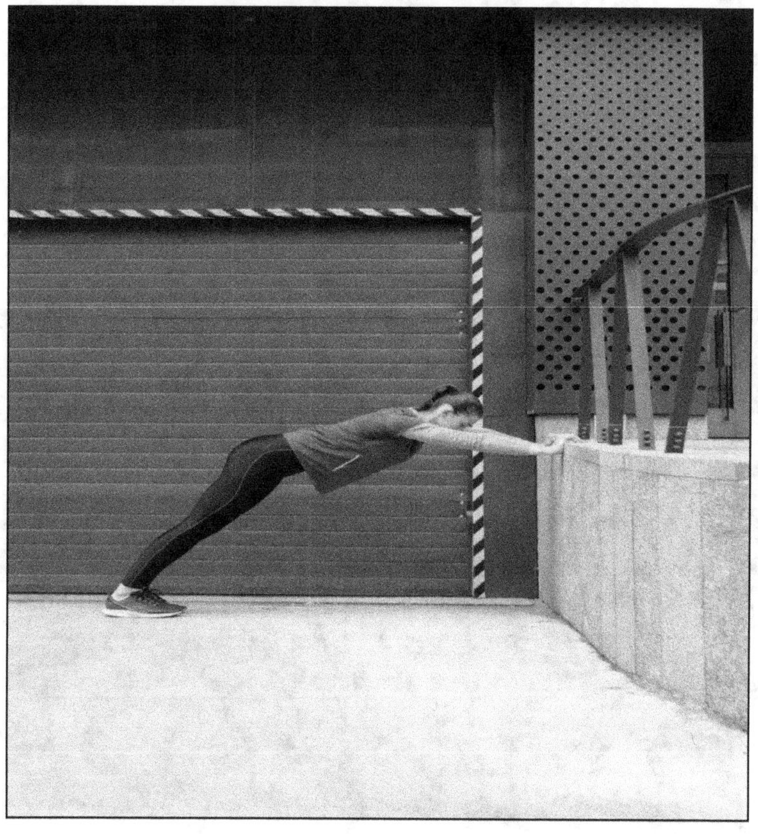

This Cover Has Been Designed From
Freepik.com

Table Of Content

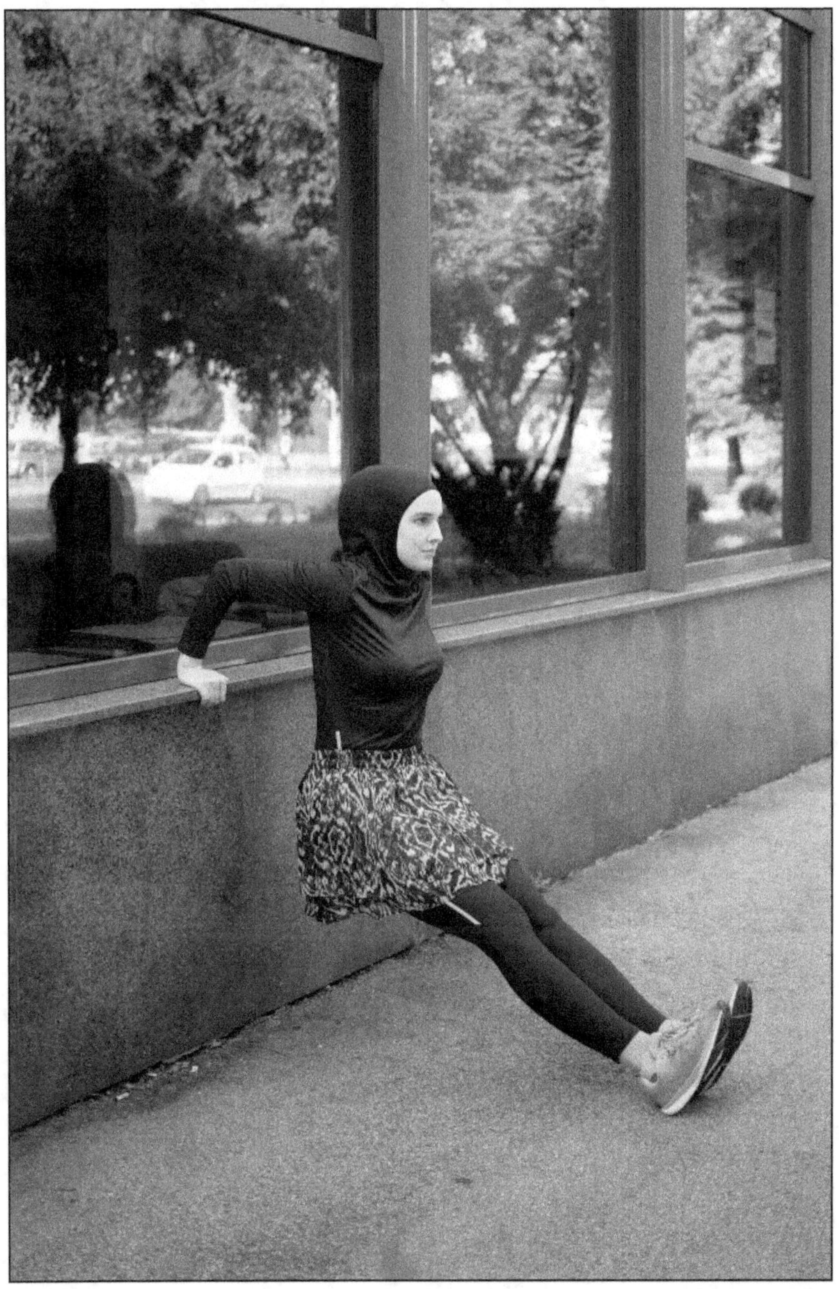

Taylor Susan. C.

Introduction

By a particular age, keeping mentally and physically fit and keeping wellness is essential, specifically for older people. This free Wall Pilates for seniors has numerous advantages, including low-impact routines, as well as secure moves to eliminate the danger of injury.

Wall Pilates is an activity that offers aid, balance, and fitness to elders and beginners. This simple and easy Pilates form promotes strength, balance, and flexibility while also relieving joint pain. Wall Pilates, when incorporated into a senior's training routine, can improve overall well-being and daily life.

This interesting post is written specifically for senior citizens. What is wall Pilates for seniors, safety considerations, safe and easy wall Pilates exercises, benefits of wall Pilates, and advice for successful wall Pilates exercises are all covered.

Wall Pilates for Seniors is an adaptation of the standard Pilates practice. During the exercise, the provided wall is used for resistance, aid, and balance. Senior Pilates workouts consist of unique positions and a series of movements that improve protection and balance.

When the body begins to degenerate, senior adults' mind-body coordination and physical capacities begin to deteriorate. As a result, problems such as joint discomfort, back pain, weight gain, increased risk of chronic diseases, and so on emerge, resulting in a lower quality of life.

With all of these issues that senior citizens face, wall Pilates exercises are a godsend. This exercise's movements are all low-impact and can be done at home with minimal equipment. Many skills are acquired as a result of this, including core strength, body alignment, body awareness, flexibility, and mobility.

So, does Wall Pilates help with weight loss? Without a doubt, YES. Individuals can enhance their general state of health by learning the ideas and qualities of wall Pilates. The simplicity of wall Pilates makes it straightforward to adapt for both elders and beginners. As a result, it may be done at home in your own time and with little equipment.

Chapter One

The Origin Of Wall Pilates

Pilates is named after the Italian physician Joseph Pilates who pioneered workout routines in the 1920s. It includes routines of motion that emphasize appropriate stance, appropriate adaptability, and stamina. It can be completed for a Revolutionary device or on an exercise mat on the ground. The Reformer employs pulleys with heightened resistance from the participant's body's weight, as well as various levels of springs.

Pilates, like yoga, promotes deep breathing. By concentrating on your breathing, you can get big results in less time. Aside from breathing, it is critical to perform regulated motions with comfort and smoothness. Pilates movements are not intended to be rigid; instead, each portion of the human body has to move in one smooth movement.

Pilates is also built with adaptations so that individuals with different types and capabilities can be physically fit while remaining safe. It is an ideal training program for older folks since it does not have the same impact on the body as other kinds of physical activity and is not as taxing on the joints as most routines. If you're wondering if Pilates is suited for you, you should think about what you want to achieve.

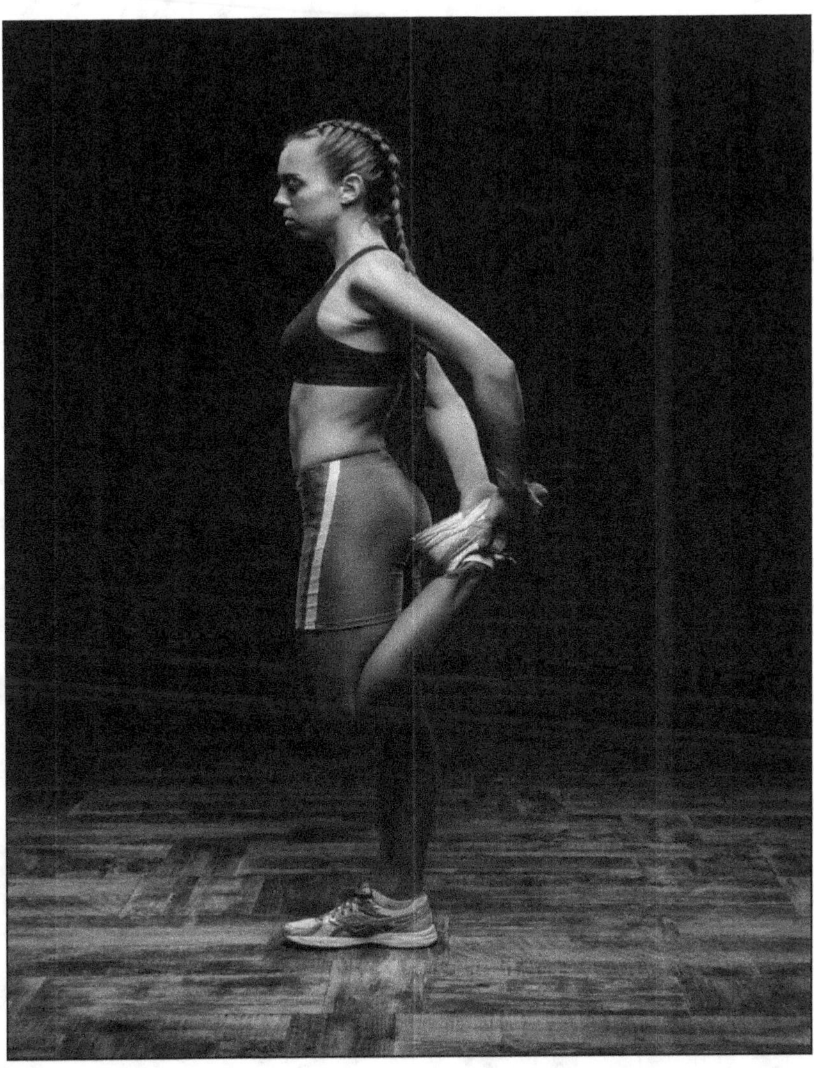

Chapter Two

Seniors' Safety Considerations

Seniors should contact their doctor or a trained healthcare expert before commencing any workout program or Wall Pilates Challenge. They will provide you with a good guideline that is ideal for Wall Pilates while keeping your health conditions in mind.

Tori Repa Wall Pilates is not the same as Wall Pilates for Seniors. Senior citizens must listen to their bodies and exercise within their limits and comfort. If certain tasks are difficult or if pain continues after a workout.

So you can make it easier by changing things like the range of motion, count, or intensity.

Cushions or props can also be used to provide additional support.

Warm-up: Preparing the body for activity lowers the chance of injury and boosts blood flow.

Breathing Technique: With controlled and deep breathing, more oxygen is absorbed by the muscles, and the back is well supported in every action due to the air in the lungs.

Rest and Hydration: 30-60 seconds of rest during exercise or between sets, as well as water intake for hydration is required to avoid overexertion and tiredness.

Better environment: There should be ample space for Wall Pilates to be practiced. Obstacles and slippery surfaces should be avoided in your workout area since they may interfere with the exercise.

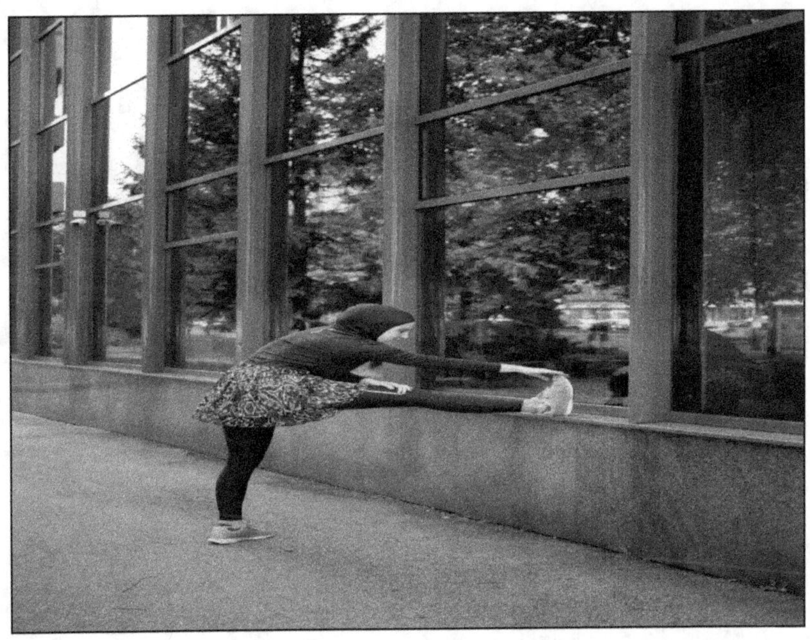

Chapter Three

Lovely Wall Pilates Rewards for Older Individuals

Pilates's physical activities are capable of providing a lot to older people. Joint discomfort, health-related issues, weariness, obesity, and other issues are common with old people. As a result of these factors, they avoid all actions that have an impact.

Nevertheless, Wall Pilates workouts are distinct in that all exercises are carried out against a wall and are adjusted to individual requirements and competencies. See More Advantages of Wall Pilates.

1. Improved physical stability and balance allow the body to be more active and agile.

2. Reduced stiffness and joint pain issues

3. Enhanced agility and range ability to move

4. Well-being of the mind and emotions

5. Improved strength in the core and posture

Wall Pilates For Seniors Over 70

Simple and safe Seniors Wall Pilates Training Guide

This collection of wall exercise routines for seniors contains wall workouts that may be done safely and readily without adequate potential harm.

Important Points to Consider for a Healthy Wall Pilates Procedure.

Having these ideas in your head, Wall Pilates may be carried out at home and is harmless and helpful for senior folks. Begin immediately with integrating Turbo The Pilates method via the gym schedule.

The Wall Pilates fitness guide/plan: A piece of Wall Pilates plan of action or chart is required to cover Wall Pilates into your regimen. You can choose from our Wall Pilates Trial chart or the best Wall Pilates regimens for elderly people mentioned already.

Choose a solid wall: The wall is one of the most vital components of Wall Pilates. A clean and polished wall can boost gym performance by giving you additional assistance and grip while exercising.

Begin with fundamental exercises: Begin with low-intensity exercise and subsequently grow. Do not engage in any strenuous or tough exercise.

Concentrate on form and control: Adapting to any physical activity takes time and practice. As a result, your workout should last 15-20 minutes. This will result in optimum structure and managerial capabilities.

Progression should be made gradually to achieve greater results and fitness while minimizing risk. The first 1-2 weeks should be spent working on form and technique. The intensity of the activity can then be increased safely.

4 Advantages of Pilates Activity

1. Pilates can help in recovery from surgical procedures such as hip replacement or knee replacement. Several of the routines can be done while reclining or sitting to help persons with restricted mobility.

Do you need any more reasons to try Pilates? Here are four more advantages.

1. The emphasis is on developing a strong core.

2. It teaches control as well as balance in a short range of motion, gradually progressing to a broader range of motion as people acquire confidence.

3. Uses breathing routines to help manage every movement, helping you to take calm, deep breaths in

and breathe out. This also has a soothing effect, which aids in stress reduction.

4. Increases versatility and breadth of motion, putting less strain on joints and allowing for smoother movements. Pilates might assist in correcting imbalances in muscles by concentrating on the way you move.

5. Aids in the treatment of a range of age-related disorders, including arthritis. Gentle mid-range movements reduce the possibility of joints collapsing while preserving the mobility around them.

These advantages aid the aging body by targeting the engine for successful exercise. The lower abdomen, backbone, glutes, thighs, and pelvic region make up the powerhouse. Need some pointers? At home, try these eight Pilates routines!

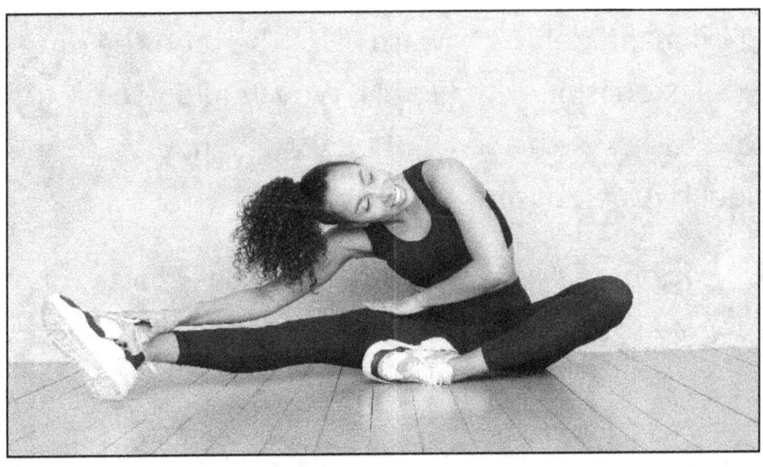

Chapter Four

Wall Pilates Materials: All You Required for Success

If you're a qualified Pilates coach contemplating opening an apartment studio or a Pilates fan who wants to get machinery for your residence, grasping the details of wall Pilates materials ought to constitute the main focus. Here's all you desire to be informed about to choose the finest wall Pilates devices for reducing body fat in your modest business or home studio.

Why Is Wall-Mounted Pilates Material More Superior?

Preparing and delving toward all of the required props for wall exercising with Pilates. Why would you pick this set of tools over the conventional ones that we frequently see utilized?

It's affordable - A Pilates program typically costs roughly the same as it would since educators must undergo intensive education and Pilates machinery, notably the reformer bed, is very costly.

In comparison, a wall Pilates unit is far less expensive. As a brand-new studio owner, you're already putting down a lot of money. Obtaining wall Pilates resources will be less expensive than reformers.

It takes up less space - Because they hang on the wall rather than lying horizontally on the floor, they make ideal apparatus for Pilates in one's house or a small studio. Provide a full-body workout; Basic Pilates has already been a core-intensive workout. However, because of the table's configuration, the workout does not put your muscles to the test as much.

In contrast, the wall Pilates apparatus is considered to put more strain on your muscles, particularly your lower body.

What is an effective wall Pilates machinery for household utilize?

As soon as it concerns determining that wall Pilates machinery is appropriate for indoor or outdoor studio utilization, the correct response usually varies by person.

a total of three primary kinds of wall components accessible on shelves nowadays.

A ladder component has boards of wood running over its entire length from the highest point to the bottom. It enables an individual to do so from varied excessive levels, increasing the intensity of the practice. Rather than springs, this component includes rubber bands.

The basic springboard component - The back is a standard wooden panel aimed at providing additional balance, particularly for powerful routines with a great deal of pulling. The wooden spring component also includes more spring connections unlike the ladder or simplistic form.

Little design - The straightforward item has a rear opening with platforms made of wood at the peak and bottom to attach to the wall. By the maker, such structures may have less or the same number of springs as the wooden component. Choose the one that most closely fits what you like.

What Machinery Should One Utilize for Wall Pilates?

If you are unable to purchase a wall component, an alternative is to try the wildly popular Wall Pilates, which is limited to four separate spaces in your residence. Below is an overview of Wall Pilates machinery that will aid make maximum benefit out of your routine.

A mat for exercising softens the impact of the rough ground on the back of your body. Resistance objects are fantastic for strengthening tissue and adding obstruction to any activity, including Pilates.

Pilates ball - The ball, such as a resistance band, contributes to the hardness of numerous conventional routines. The noise object is beneficial for Pilates routines that emphasize the muscles of the downward region (legs, waist, and glutes), wall movement, and squats as well as flexion and lengthening motions.

Ankle weights may aid you in strengthening courage, most notably in the lower body by offering pressure.

Finally, what is the greatest wall Pilates machinery?

Some of the crucial Wall Pilates instruments for studios are user-friendly wall units and well-padded yoga mats. The wall module is ideal for numerous routines. If you'd like to practice wall Pilates within your house but are unable to purchase the wall unit, a decent yoga mat, and any wall in your house would suffice. Weights, resistance rubber, and balls are nice additions but not required.

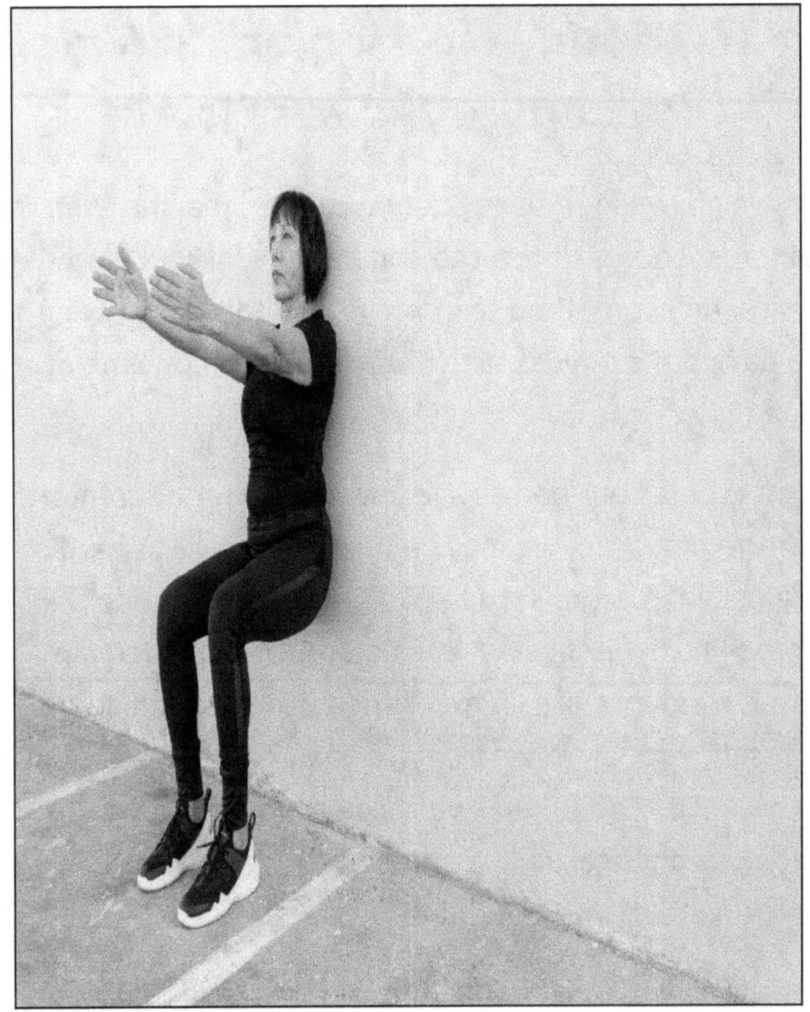

Chapter Five

Wall Routines for Seniors: A Simple Procedure to Stay Strong

As we grow older, our system weakens, making even the quickest chores difficult to complete. Workout is a great and simplest method to improve our bodies, allowing us to navigate everyday activities with more convenience and fewer aches.

However, as our bodies age and encounter discomfort for the first time, we may be unable to work as hard as we once did. Here's where wall workouts for elders come in. Low-impact wall regimens for the elderly in one's residence are an excellent method to bring oneself, your elderly parents, or older relatives back into fitness. They additionally provide a wonderful way to increase physical ability, enabling aging persons to remain more autonomous.

Here's all you must understand about these routines, as well as an array of basic regular wall routines for the elderly to boost wellness and build tough muscles.

What Are Wall Workouts for Aging People?

Wall movements for elderly people, also known as wall Pilates, are an alternate method for people over 65 to get in shape and enhance their overall wellness. The activities use a wall for more assistance, allowing older folks to complete activities that they would not normally be capable of accomplishing.

In contrast to regularly working out, Pilates wall routines for the elderly involve calm, deliberate moves instead of quick, intense activities. This makes the workouts faster to learn, engage, and do, as well as healthier for numerous aging individuals' speed and durable abilities.

Seniors are far more inclined to adhere to such an exercise schedule than those who need a faster speed and greater strength. This book is your accelerated ticket to long-term weight loss! With just a few swipes, you can personalize your exercise path and maximize your results!

However, a few classes are more appropriate for those over 65, specifically those who are novice fitness novices drills include:

Aerobic activities include trekking, swimming, biking, and dancing.

Strengthening your muscles encompasses the majority of wall workouts for aging people. A meta-analysis issued by the scientific journal Frontiers in Psychological found that physical activity is more beneficial than conventional aerobics.

Studies discovered that resistance drills are quite effective at increasing motion, quickly, and power in the lower limbs while simultaneously lessening trunk fat. In reality, integrating strengthening with aerobics is proven to enhance sitting and stretches, elbow, knee, and shoulder extension and stretching, power and fatty tissue mass, useful reach scrutiny, 30-cycle chair sitting evaluation, and 6-minute strolling assessments, as well as reflection of body function.

Yoga, martial arts, and wall-widening activities are all good instances of balance and state of movement. Posture and movement drills can assist those over 65 enhance their equilibrium, peace of mind, interaction, accessibility, and assurance. All of these will contribute to a higher and greater standard of life.

How Might a 65-Year-Old Remain in Shape?

There's no age restriction for getting into form. If you're 65 or older and want to get in form. Below are a few suggestions and procedures for assisting you on this enjoyable, demanding, and extremely gratifying path.

Procedure your workout trip.

The initial procedure in every fitness quest is to get up and work out. As discussed in the last phase, we have numerous activities to start from. Go with one and try it; if you don't think it's for you, try a different thing. Continue till you discover anything you truly cherish and like doing. Remember that working out provides more than just physical pleasures.

Studies have shown that frequent working out in elderly persons is connected with better immune system, behavioral wellness, feelings, thoughts, a positive social life, higher standards of life, and overall wellness.

Remain consistent.

Always remember that uniformity is of greater significance than motivation. It's sometimes simple to summon up the drive to hit the gym or get up from your sofa for a 30-minute at-home drill. Nevertheless, if you encourage yourself to persevere despite your drive, you will most likely achieve your objective of getting fit.

Begin with lower/simpler workouts.

The secret to an amazing fitness regimen is to do something you enjoy while simultaneously pacing yourself. Taking action excessively at once may cause you to quit your regimen objective more quickly than you might imagine.

For those new to working out, we recommend starting with simple routines like wall Pilates routines for the elderly, yoga, martial arts, or simply strolling. Such instances necessitate a more gradual rate, which is ideal for easing you into a continuous pattern of drills.

Enhance your level of effort.

Yes, you have to begin slowly. Nevertheless, after a while of performing similar activities, one's the body may become accustomed to the exertion and begin to stall.

Once you reach a point where you will never again experience gain in weight (if underweight), loss of weight (if overweight), or body composition adjustments. you avoid this, ensure that you up the level of sensitivity of how your every week basis effort translates to more stress, additional energy expended, and, eventually, more muscular growth.

Find a community.

A 2017 study published in the American Magazine of Our Way of Life Medical Sciences discovered that humans thrive in communal situations. This research emphasizes the link between public contact and things that can aid individuals preserve an appropriate body mass index (BMI), regulate blood sugars, enhance cancer survival, reduce death from cardiovascular disease and depressive signs, alleviate post-

Traumatic Stress Disorder signs, and enhance wellness.

In light of this research, it is best to find an organization or community of individuals to routine with. Moreover, completing simple wall routines at home will produce the required effects, but joining a group of individuals with similar goals will aid you in maintaining discipline.

It may additionally render how you train routines more enjoyable and bring you new fun routines that you might not have thought of normally.

What Are Five Training Sessions for Individuals Over 50?

Some routines that are ideal for people over the age of fifty include:

Walking

This is the coolest workout that everyone can complete, no matter of time, location, or age. Begin by encouraging oneself to get outside for a comfortable period every day. According to a 2011 study, the average amount of steps taken by healthy older persons per day ranged from 2,000 to 9,000. You can do far more than you may realize.

Core workouts

A robust core is required to elevate the way you stand and to equilibrium, and stability of the lower vertebrae, and increased flexibility. Sitting ups, crunches, and wall planks are all basic wall routines for seniors. They also make wonderful upgrades to your wall routines for flat tummy application.

Strength daily: Since we become older, we decrease muscular mass and performance. Strength training slows or stops this procedure by assisting in tissue preservation and growth. Begin with lighter weight and higher reps per set.

Yoga and Pilates are effective types of practice for developing a strong core, equilibrium, and suppleness. You can meet up to take programs or find internet-based things that enable you to conduct such drills at home.

Dancing can be a significant impact or gentle session, based on your preference. Irrespective of your preference, it is a pleasant way to relax for a few hrs and eliminate calories.

What Are the Top Wall Drills for Older People?

Below are a few basic wall drills for the elderly to do at home:

1. Wall Push-ups

These are an excellent upper-body routine that grows muscle and strengthens the upper body.

1. Stand a few inches from the wall, legs spread out.

2. Spread both hands widely on the wall at the level of the shoulders. If it is difficult for you to feel a wall, move closer.

3. Progressively bend your elbows and lean your body against the wall till your nose nearly meets it. Maintain a firm core (draw your abdomen closer to the spine), an erect back, and elbows bent at approximately 45°.

4. Delicately return to the initial stance.

5. Carry out 5 to 10 sets per set.

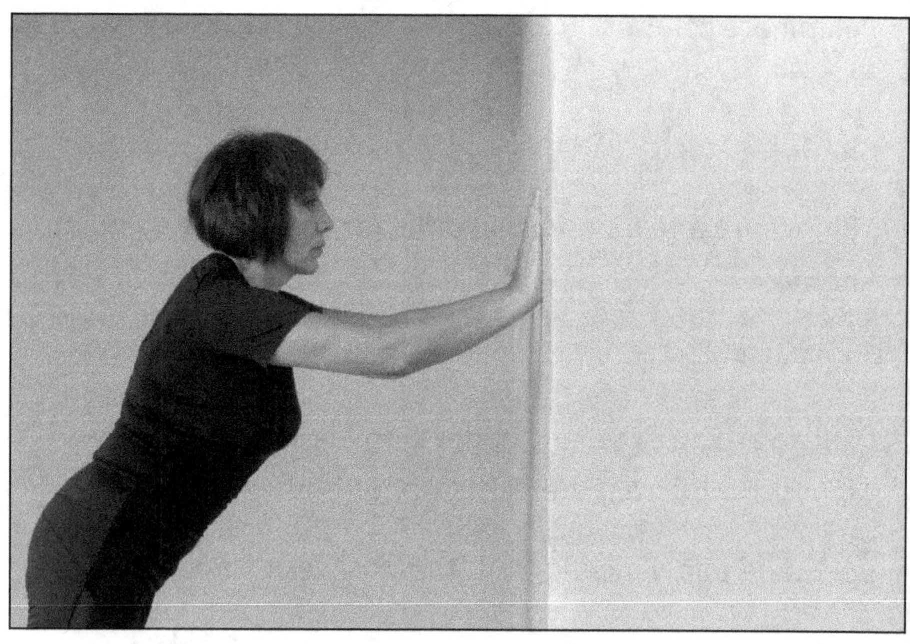

2. Standing Wall Planks

Planks are a fantastic practice for ability in the core, equilibrium, and stance.

1. Begin by sitting upright and in front of the wall. Straighten your hands, crook your elbows, and rest your hands opposite the wall. Your elbows ought to be high above the shoulders, and your palms should be in a direction up toward the wall.

2. Retain robust shoulders and gradually lean into your forearms. Tuck your elbows into the wall to avoid the blades of your shoulder from jutting out.

3. Take a few steps away from the wall and maintain your body erect and your core firm.

4. This positions your body at an incline. Make sure your hips and buttocks do not bulge out behind you.

5. Hold the pose for a maximum of a few moments.

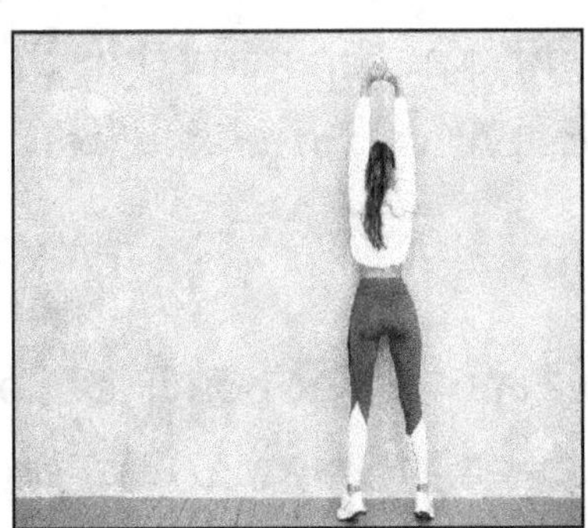

3. Walking From Heel to Toe

Heel-to-toe walking is a wonderful way to boost your agility and balance. The activity is typically performed in the absence of the use of a wall, however, if you can't do it In the absence of it, this is a fantastic place to start.

1. Stay with your side at a distance of one arm from a wall. Place your nearest hand on the wall.

2. Put your right leg just in front of the left one, with the heel of your right leg touching the tops of your left foot's toes.

3. Put the left foot in the center of your right leg, with the pressure on the back of your heel. Then move all of your weight onto your toes.

4. Make this procedure with the left foot. Walk in this manner. For 20 reps

5. The hand nearest to the wall may gently skim it and not bear your weight. Keep in mind that the hand is only on the wall in the event you lose balance.

4. Wall Back Leg Lifts

This is a successful team lower-body development routine that focuses on the hips, glutes, and feet.

1. Sit an arm's length from a wall.

2. Move both arms forward the wall while engaging your abdominal muscles.

3. Carefully lift your right foot directly back, without bending your knees or pointing your toes.

4. Sustain the 'kick back' stance for a brief period while gradually releasing your leg.

5. Do this between eight and twelve times on the reverse leg to do a single set, then change and continue on the left.

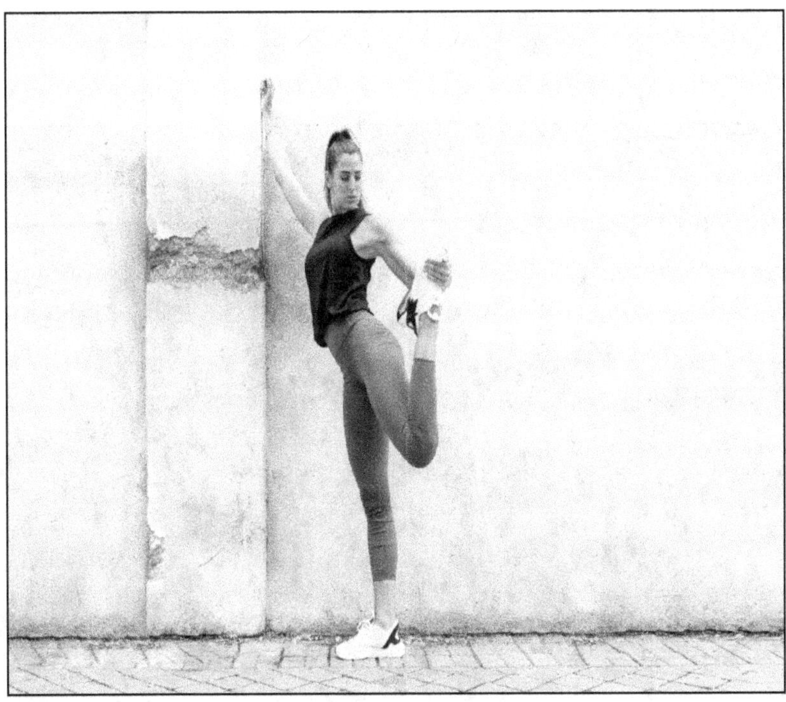

5. Wall-Toe raises

This is a different wonderful lower-body practice that works your legs and is outstanding for equilibrium.

1. Stand around a few inches distant from a wall.

2. Straighten the hands and direct them towards the wall. Tighten their cores.

3. Raise yourself onto your feet as high as feasible, then gradually bring yourself back below.

5. Strive not to place your back too much ahead against the wall.

6. Carry out 15–20 times.

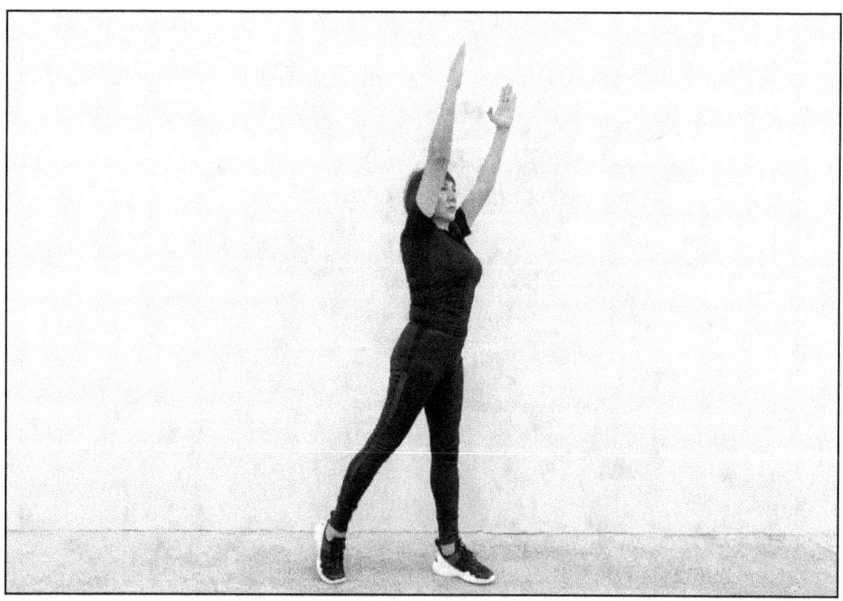

6. Wall Side Leg Lifts

Side leg raises, like back leg lifts, are a cool workout for your bottom leg. They develop the outer legs, hips, and buttocks while increasing hip movement and ability.

1. Stand within a distance of an arm from a wall. Raise both arms, forcing them against the wall while Maintaining your abdominal muscles connected.

2. Carefully elevate your right foot in the opposite direction. Maintain your back upright, toes sticking on, and gaze upward.

3. Maintain the lifted stance for a moment while slowly decreasing your leg to the floor.

4. Carry out 12 to 15 rounds of this procedure then swapping feet and restarting the workout.

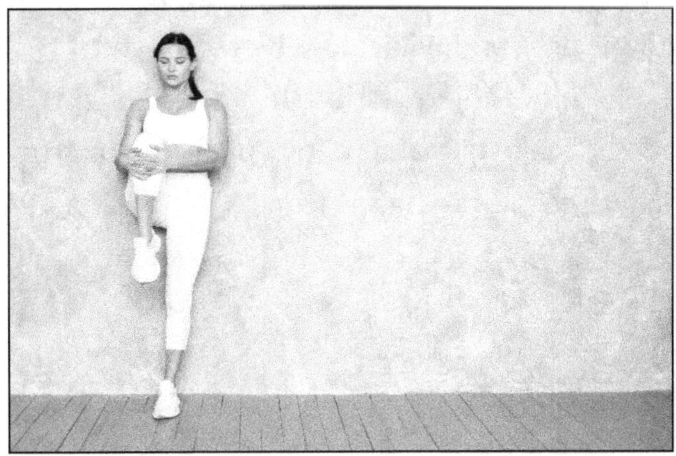

Chapter Six

6 Wall Pilates Ab Classes Practice You ought to Add To Your daily grind

For countless exercisers, abs are an elusive muscle area that is typically viewed as an avatar of perfect bodily condition. By using this technique, these specific muscles are exalted at the cost of other equally vital areas of muscle that contribute to our good posture, equilibrium, and general strength.

Having a chiseled six-pack, on the other hand, necessitates not only continuous workouts but also a range of activities that improve various portions of your core. However, a wall Pilates ab workout isn't completely out of the question. It is an excellent approach to make use of a readily available instrument for effective core training.

Is Wall Pilates Useful for Abs?

Yes, wall Pilates might allow tighten your abs and make them more apparent. Using wall training sessions for abs for both newbies and veterans ensures:

1. You're Using Numerous Muscle Sections

Wall Pilates does not separate the muscles of the tummy, instead, it stimulates the use of numerous muscular groups. several people are unaware that their "abs" are made up of several muscles and represent just one element of the system that makes up the body's core. The transverse Abdominis, obliques, and Rectus Abdominis are the muscles of the belly.

Wall Pilates routines address all the aforementioned muscles, assisting you in achieving a better core. A more well-rounded and thorough physical activity arises from this kind of complete strategy.

Working your abs further develops muscles that provide support in your back and waist, providing greater stability and perhaps lowering your chance of injury. Furthermore, using many muscles at the same time may enhance calorie burn, which assists in fat reduction gradually, causing those abs stronger.

2. You're Boosting Your Body Sensitivity Wall Pilates

movements demand accuracy and oversight, forcing you to grow more mindful of your body's balance. This increased sense of self, or sense of balance, is useful for maintaining the correct posture and avoiding accidents.

When you exercise your abs actively and emphasize balancing your body with the wall, you are more inclined to trigger the more profound and frequently overlooked abs muscles, leading to a more distinct and powerful core.

3. You are boosting your solid foundation.

Integrating the wall into your Pilates physical activity creates outside resistance, forcing those core muscles to operate harder. This additional difficulty may result in broadened ab endurance and balance.

In addition, the wall gives tactile input, aiding you with keeping good form and position, which is critical for working the abs successfully.

4. You're Developing Wall Flexibility and Mobility Pilates

Physical activity frequently incorporates dynamic movement, which could strengthen your balance and mobility. Enhanced flexibility may help you do ab-targeting exercise routines with greater results, and better movement might assist you in preventing wounds. Pilates gives a mix of both endurance and flexibility, that's needed in building a well-defined and functioning core.

5. You're Making Use of a Simple and Versatile Tool

The wall is a simple piece of equipment that can be used in a variety of ways to target your abs. It's a multipurpose instrument that can accommodate people of all fitness levels. Beginners may utilize the wall for support and direction while doing exercises, while more skilled users can use it for increased resistance or to execute more difficult variants.

6. You're modifying Up the Way You Exercise

By including wall activities into the regimen, you add diversity to your workouts, which not only keeps them interesting but pushes your muscles in new ways. This is significant because muscular adaptation might result in a fitness plateau.

By continually modifying your routines, you increase your chances of growing and seeing those desired abs sooner.

Does Wall Pilates Assist for the Decrease of Stomach Fat?

Yes, wall Pilates might assist you in losing belly fat. It constitutes a full-body leverage that burns calories just like any other sort of physical activity. Despite it may not burn the same calories as high-intensity activities like running or cycling, it does add to general calorie burn.

More significantly, Pilates, particularly wall Pilates, may aid in the development of lean muscular mass.

How Is the Belly Fat Wall Activity Performed?

Wall Pilates sessions for belly fat demand you to use your ab muscles in opposition to the stress of the wall. This is performed by performing a series of tummy muscle-targeting routines to become fit, focusing mainly on the rectus abdominis, transversal abdominis, and obliquely.

1. Wall Planks

When it comes to one of the best Abs training wall Pilates is highly rated and recommended. This exercise is easy to carry out, and it plays a great role in targeting the Rectus Abdominis. The wall plank workout came to be from the traditional plank exercise of Pilates. This has to do with the use of wall in your environment to participate in this training session.

This also helps in the core training activities because of its importance in engaging numerous tissues, and muscles in our body systems.

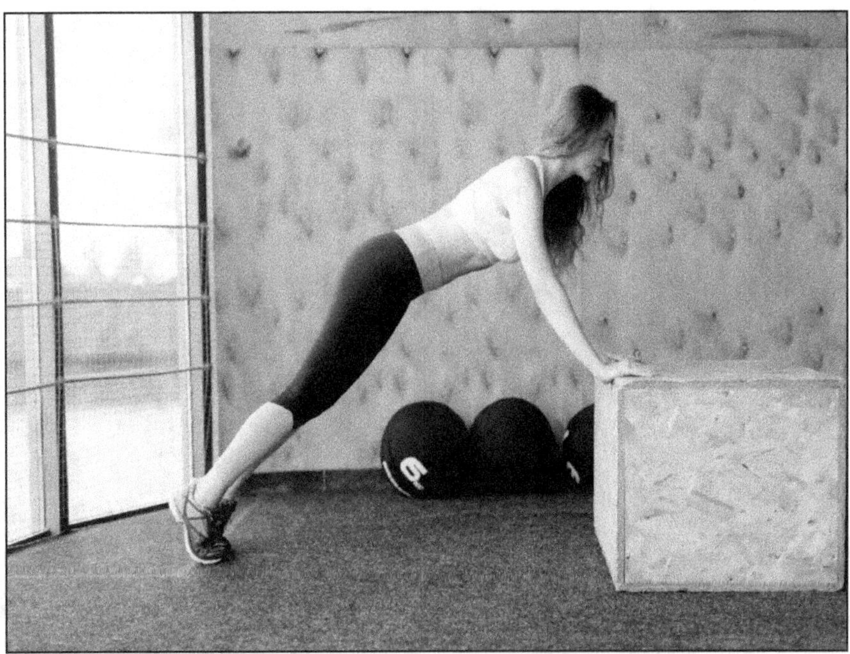

Procedure:

1. First, pick any spot or position of your choice, via any wall in your room for people who will love to do this beautiful exercise in their rooms.

2. Place your two hands on the wall with your shoulder width apart.

3. Then, you need to move your feet backward until you get the plank position angled toward your wall.

4. You need to make sure that your Abs engages while doing this and also create a straight

posture or line from your head down to your feet.

5. Maintain this training position for 30-40 seconds to a minute and so on depending on your ability and your desire.

6. Take a break and repeat this procedure for any set or amount of time you love.

2. Wall Push-ups

As its name implies it's the type of wall Pilates exercise that is done on the wall which got its name from the traditional push-ups. The wall Push-ups is a very lovely, and simple exercise that can be carried out at your convenient time.

One alluring thing about this exercise is that's beginner-friendly and focuses on your upper body and abs. The resistance from the wall, paired with the engagement of the core makes it a very good wall Pilates for tummy fat novice's training.

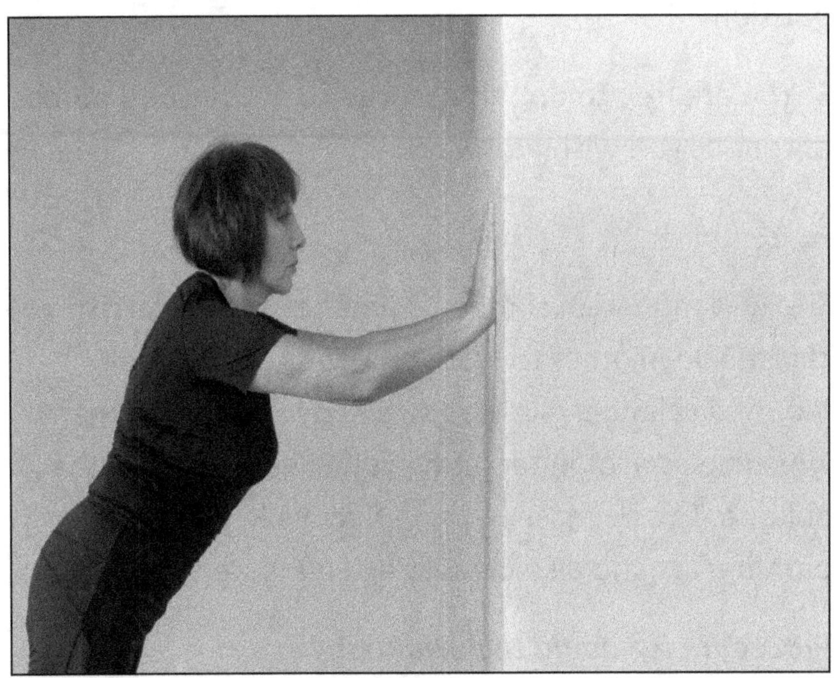

Procedure for doing this workout:

1. Stand erect and face your wall.

2. Then, you need to put your hands on your chest level, and a little bit wider than your shoulder width separation.

3. Keep your legs firmly on the floor, and lower your chest closer to the wall as you bend your elbows.

4. Engage your Abs, and make sure that your body is in a straight posture as you bring yourself back to the initial position.

5. You are free to do this exercise to any desired number of rounds you wish and want.

3. Wall Mountain Climber

The wall mountain climber is another great exercise you can still do in other to work on your Abs. The wall mountain climber is mixed with a dynamic movement which helps a lot in targeting your Abs, especially the oblique. This exercise is very effective in terms of burning fats and also in building your core strength.

Procedure for doing this workout:

1. Stand and face your wall.

2. Then, you ought to get into a high plank position with your palms on the wall.

3. Try to engage your Abs as you bring one of your knees towards your chest.

4. Take your feet back to the ground as you switch the other feet.

5. This exercise can be done at any desired number and rounds.

4. Wall Sit With Your Abs Twist

The wall sit with the Abs twist pairs an isometric workout i.e. (the wall sit) and the dynamic movement (Abs twist). This exercise helps effectively for the building of Abs and glutes, making it a very good wall Pilates exercise for both the glutes and the core.

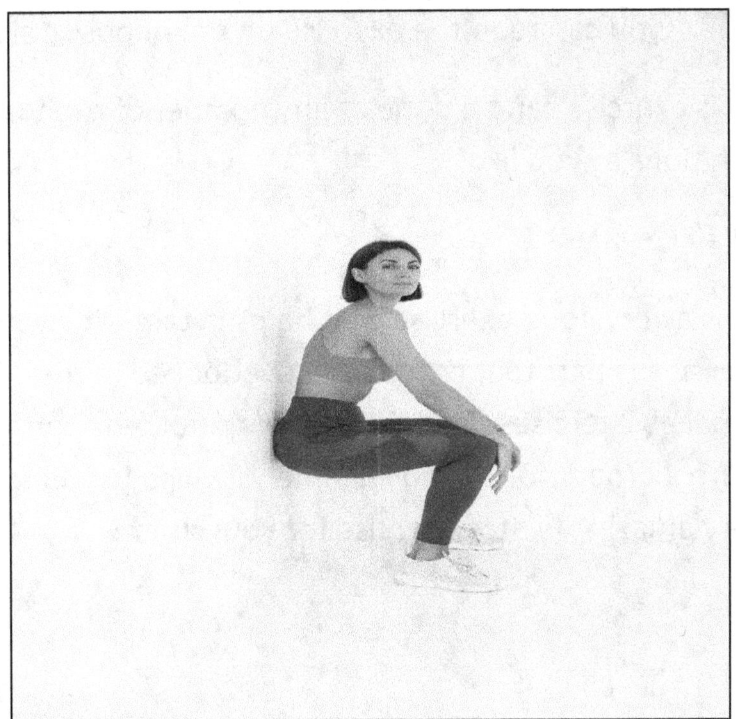

Procedure In To do this exercise:

1. Stand in a position where your back is facing your wall.

2. Then, bring yourself down or lower your body into a squat position with your thighs erect to the ground.

3. Put your hand on your hips.

4. Try to engage your Abs as you twist your torso to one side, then return to the center.

5. Then, you can redo the exercise on the opposite side.

6. This exercise can be done at any number of rounds or repetitions as you like.

5. Wall Leg Raise

This is a very good exercise that helps in targeting your lower abs, a part that is normally overlooked in the normal ab exercises. By doing this workout, you can ensure a proper form, and alignment, which is said to be a very amazing Pilates exercise for your tummy.

Step of doing this workout:

1. Lie on your mat, and raise your legs to the wall in front of you.

2. Put your hands on your sides.

3. Try and engage your Abs as you raise your hips off the ground, and push your feet into the wall.

4. Then, you need to lower your hips back down on your mat.

5. You can do this exercise at any desired number of repetitions.

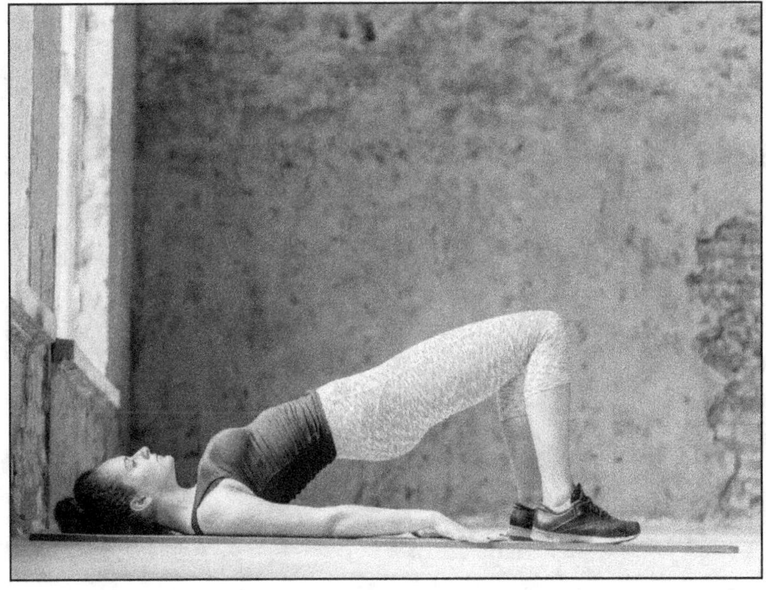

6. Wall Bridge

This is another great wall Pilates exercise that helps in targeting the deeper core muscles. It's a good exercise for beginners because of how easy and simple the exercise is in toning the Abs.

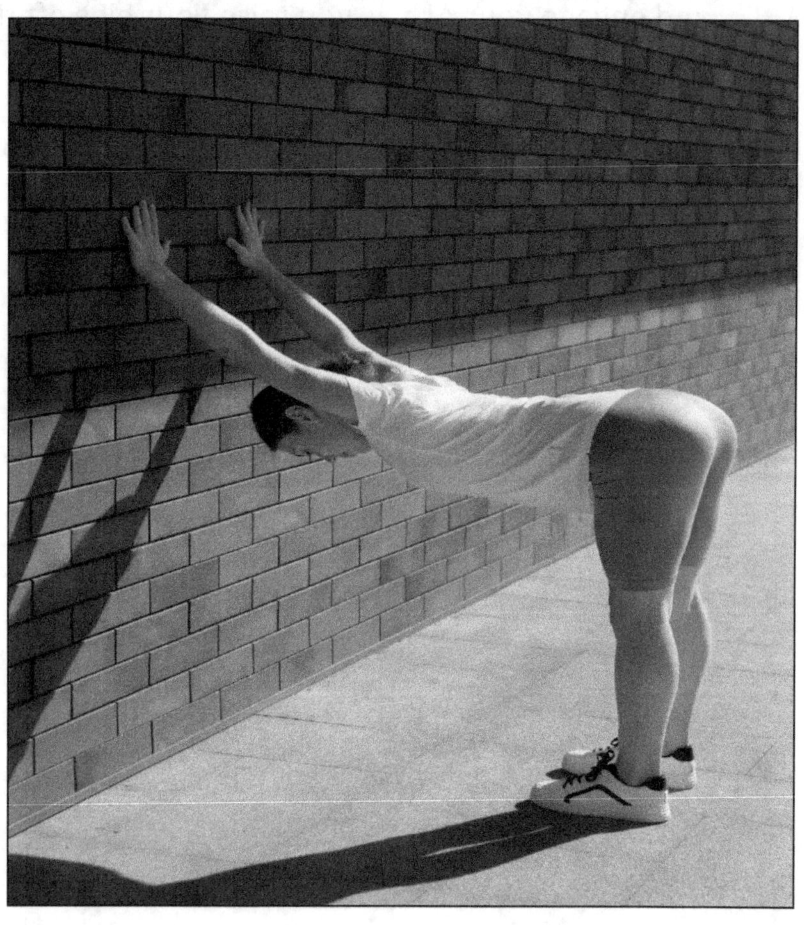

Steps in doing this workout:

1. Lie On your back with your knees bent and legs flat on the wall.

2. Put your hand on your sides.

3. Exhale and try lifting your hips off the wall, and make sure that you are pressing your feet on the wall.

4. Inhale and gently lower your hips back to the floor at the initial starting point.

5. You are free to carry out this exercise at any desired number of repetitions.

Can I do Pilates daily?

Yes, you could perform Pilates regularly as long as you remain mindful of how your entire the system reacts and doesn't overtrain. For novices, we suggest beginning with a two-to-three-times-a-week wall Pilates ab exercise for beginners and eventually building to a daily program. This gradual approach will enable your body to adjust to the new motions and effort, reducing the risk of injury.

You can indulge in wall Pilates for abdominal and glutes or various wall routines for abs daily if you're intermediate or developed, but you'll need to alter the duration and emphasis of the physical activity to prevent excessive exercise and plateauing.

To properly target various muscle areas, you may rotate among light wall training sessions for fat loss and tougher core training, such as abdominal movements.

Regardless of having discovered that Pilates is a low-impact exercise, overworking is inevitable. Over-training symptoms are weariness, poor performance, elevated resting heartbeat, and difficulty falling asleep. If you see any of the above signs, take a day or two off and adapt how you train correctly.

How Come I Can't Tone My Stomach?

If you're not seeing improvements after completing wall Pilates abdominal exercises every day, you might be committing one or more of the following errors:

You're Not Eating a Healthy Diet

You won't notice substantial effects no matter how often you work out if your food isn't balanced and healthy. Excess fat may obscure muscle definition if you eat too many processed, high-sugar, or high-fat meals.

You are not properly hydrating.

Hydration is critical for general health, including metabolic function and fat reduction. If you don't drink enough water, your body may retain water, giving you a bloated look.

You're Not Including Other Types of Exercise

While Pilates is great for core strength and toning, combining it with cardio and strength training may aid in total fat reduction and muscle growth, allowing for obvious ab definition.

You're not switching up the way you train.

A regular habit might force your body to settle in, leading to a plateau. To keep your muscles activated, try to vary your activities and create new difficulties.

You're Not Paying Attention to Form

Form and alignment are critical in Pilates. You may not be targeting your abs as successfully as you believe if your execution is poor.

You Aren't Getting A Good Night's

Rest days are critical for muscle healing and development. Overexercising without enough rest might stymie the growth of and result in weariness or injury.

You're Not Considering Stress Management

High levels of stress may cause hormonal abnormalities that encourage fat accumulation, especially in the abdominal region. Stress management practices, such as meditation or wall yoga positions, may help with general health and fitness growth.

You have unrealistic expectations.

Everyone's body reacts differently to exercise, and noticeable effects take time to appear. You may get disheartened if your expectations are unreasonable. Be patient, and persistent, and concentrate on improving strength and flexibility rather than merely appearances.

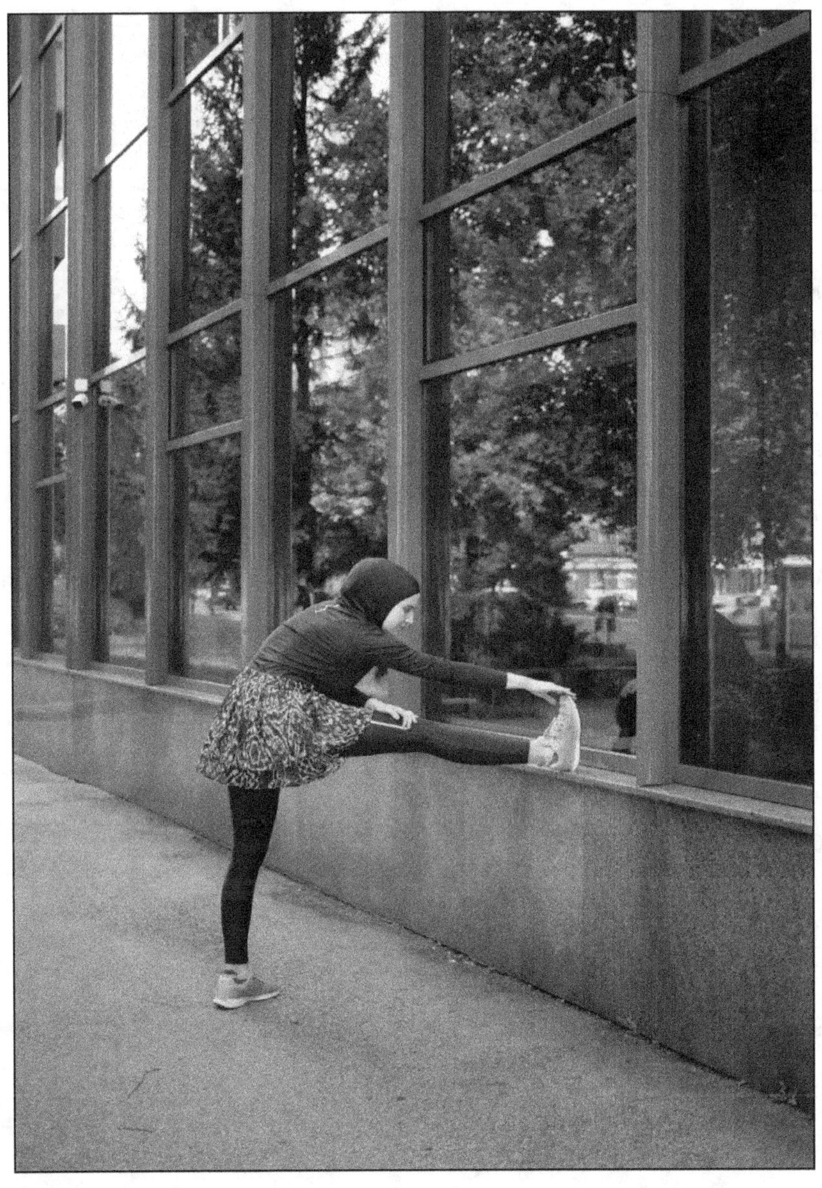

Chapter Seven

A Brief Overview for Newbies to Wall Pilates.

Pilates is most commonly done on a mat. Focused routines along with lengthy breathing may aid you bolster your core, enhance your balance, and stretch more. This technique alone may significantly boost your body's general endurance and rigidity.

When you integrate the resistance and aid of a wall into your Pilates workout, you are anticipating a completely transforming encounter. Wall Pilates may aid you not solely in stimulating certain muscle groups like the glutes, but also optimize your technique and overall efficiency.

With this in mind, in this wall Pilates for buttocks guide, we'll walk you through a variety of movements designed to be easy enough for beginners yet tough enough to produce obvious results.

What's the contrast between Pilates and Wall Pilates?

The gap between Pilates and Wall Pilates is the machinery, specifically the usage of a wall. While typical Pilates routines rely on your body fat and gravity for obstruction, wall Pilates adds another aspect by taking advantage of the assistance and rigidity of a wall.

This provides for a more focused and precise workout while also offering extra assistance for those who battle with stability or good form.

Does Wall Pilates Make You Curvier?

If you have genetically predisposed curves, wall Pilates can help to augment and define them. While it may not significantly alter your body form, it can help tone and bolster your muscles, resulting in a more distinct and sculpted impression.

Note: Because genetics play a crucial effect on body shape, Wall Pilates may not produce the same results as someone else. Nonetheless, continuous wall Pilates leverage undoubtedly boosts your entire muscle tone and definition.

Can wall Pilates aid in the development of your curves?

Wall It is delightful for shaping the glutes, and the tissue in your backside. By exercising them in specialized drills, you may elevate and develop them.

A wall Pilates routine for curves comprises:

1. Wall Squat

This is a very effective workout that concentrates the hamstring, glutes, and quadriceps.

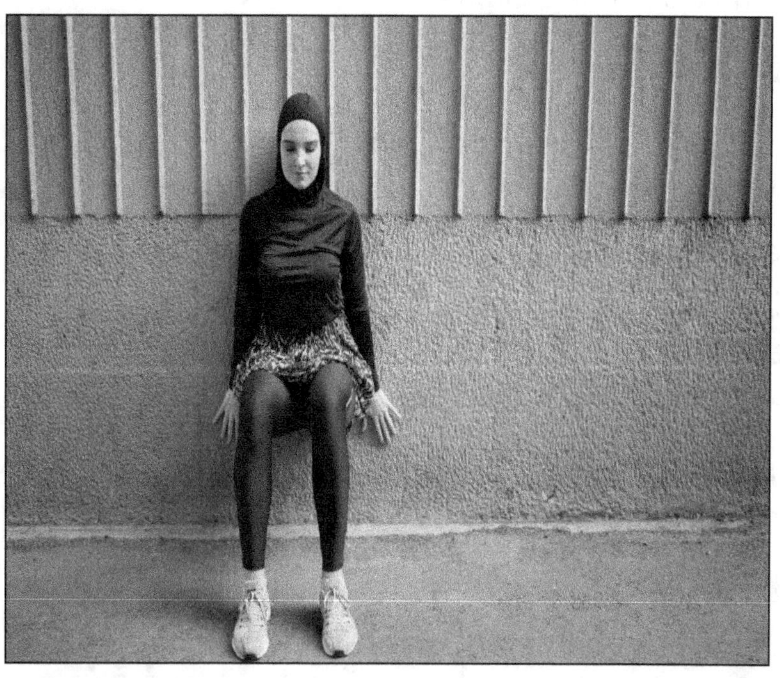

To carry out these daily drills:

1. Place your back on the wall in your room or any conducive place as you stand erect.

2. Make sure that your feet are two inches or feet away from the wall.

3. Recreate the Squat pose as you bring your body lower to a point that your knees are 90 degrees bent.

4. Stay in this recreated pose for about a minute as you engage your glutes.

5. Add more pressure to your heels as you press them on the ground. Return the your initial pose.

6. Do this drill for 9-16 times.

2. Wall Bridge

Here is another outstanding workout that will help you build your curves. To carry

This routine all you have to do is:

1. Lay on the floor with your legs on the wall.

2. Slowly raise your hips, to a straight line that runs from your knees down to your shoulder.

3. Maintain this position for a few moments as you engage your core and glutes.

4. Bring yourself back to the initial stance via the floor.

5. Do this workout 9-16 times.

3. Wall Side Leg Lifts

This is another outstanding exercise you shouldn't overlook. It focuses on the hip abductor muscle, which comprises the gluteus mediums and minims.

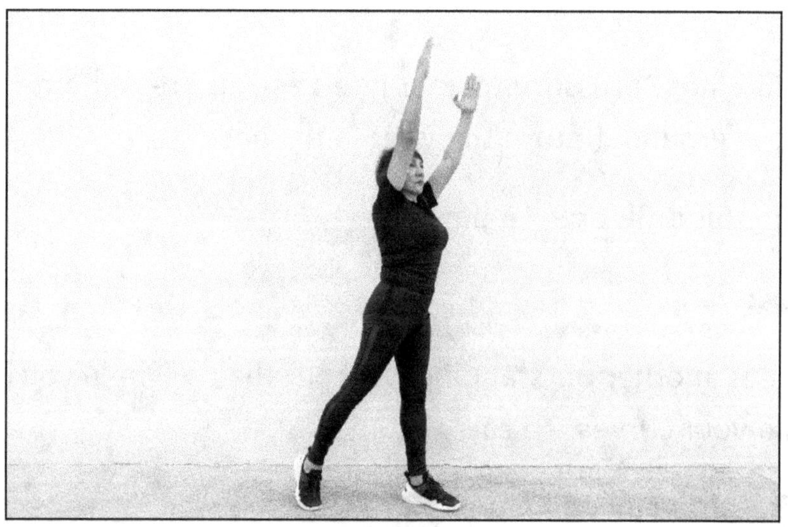

To proceed with this routine:

1. Stand still with your side on the wall in your room, with one hand on the wall to aid your balance.

2. Lift your legs out to the side, making it straight.

3. Try as much as possible to engage your core, and glutes muscles as you lift and lower your legs.

4. Do this 9-14 times on each side.

4. Wall Sit with leg lift

Here is another fantastic workout for your hip flexor, glutes, and quadriceps. To recreate these drills all you have to do is:

1. Sit against the wall in your room with your legs width apart, and ensure that your knees are at 90 degrees.

2. Lift the left or right legs off the floor by extending at the knees, to a point that it's straight.

3. Stay in this position for a few moments and lower yourself.

4. Switch legs as you carry out this daily drill 10-14 times.

Chapter Eight

FAQs

How Can I Practice Wall Workout at Home?

The simplest approach to perform the aforementioned wall workouts for elders at home is to merely begin. That is it. However, to ensure that you are as safe as feasible when working out, you might want to think about the following:

Have supervision - If you have mobility, vision, or balance concerns, it may be beneficial to have someone observe you if you fall over or something else happens.

It is not a good idea to train out on a full stomach. Eat something light, like a banana or an apple, at least 30 minutes before trying the activities listed above. It is not a good idea to train out on a full stomach. Eat something light, like a banana or an apple, at least 30 minutes before trying the activities listed above.

Find a soft area on which to sit or lie down - wall exercises are typically performed standing up, but can also be done lying down. We recommend using a soft yoga or workout mat for those activities that need you to be on the ground. It is also advisable to keep a sturdy chair nearby in case you must be seated down and rest.

Drink water - staying hydrated during your workout is essential. You can drink simple water or add fruit to it for more flavor. Pace yourself and try to start small. Do not let your excitement cause you to overwork yourself, as doing too much too soon may result in injury.

Are Wall Activities Appropriate for Those Over 65?

Indeed, they are. Wall practice for the feet, core, and upper body is shown to develop bones, enhance motor skills, raise vitality, and aid in mental abilities in older people.

How Can Elderly Training at Home?

The finest suggestions for elder at-home workouts are: Have a defined workspace; it doesn't have to be large. A space large enough to accommodate a yoga mat and allow you to move freely in a circle is acceptable. A separate place will enable you to concentrate on your training without interruptions.

Have a plan - a fixed weekly (or daily) workout regimen with particular workouts will allow you to jump right into the training without wasting time.

Have realistic goals; nothing kills the motivation to exercise faster than unrealistic aspirations. You will not notice any modifications in the first week. You're unlikely to notice any significant modifications in a month. Changes can take between 2 and 3 months to become apparent. Remember this while you work toward your goals.

What Is Recommended Training for Aged Parents?

Fitness classes are not gender or age-specific. You can accomplish anything as long as you work on your fitness and cardiovascular health, and stay safe to avoid injury. However, for novices, I prescribe simple physical activities such as walking, swimming, cycling, light strength training, Taichi, and even chair and wall Pilates routines for older people. These activities do not demand a lot of strength and may be done at a slower rate, making them a great place to begin for elders.

Conclusion

Overall, wall routines are an excellent way for elders to commence practicing. They are slow, regulated, and simple to perform, and they offer several positive health effects. These workouts may offer older persons a variety of advantages; including enhanced immunity, mental health, balance, and muscle strength. If you're searching for a regimen that can assist you consider some of the workouts listed above and build from there.

www.ingramcontent.com/pod-product-compliance
Lightning Source LLC
Chambersburg PA
CBHW070721260726
48660CB00007B/2667